"This is an intense, personal story of a woman's lifelong struggle to overcome the obstacles resulting from epilepsy beginning in childhood; her accomplishments in the face of adversity are uplifting.

As physicians we do not often get to see illness from the patient's perspective; this book provides that opportunity."

– Dr. Norman Abramson

First Edition
2017

ISBN 978-1-943492-29-9 (case bound)
ISBN 978-1-943492-24-4 (soft cover)

Book and cover design by **designpanache**

ELM GROVE PUBLISHING
San Antonio, Texas, USA
www.elmgrovepublishing.com

My Epi•Center

Epilepsy: A Woman's Point of View

EGP

Shelley Kobelsky

"The safest place during an earthquake would be in a stationary store" – *George Carlin*

(The same could be said for a seizure!) – *SK*

"Bombs don't kill people, explosions do." – *unknown**

(Again, the same is true of seizures!) – *SK*

"I'm like a computer, rebooting back to consciousness after a seizure (hopefully)." – *SK*

Foreword

The important question is: "How am I still breathing and functioning to be able to tell my story, calling myself an author?" A top concern for those with epilepsy is how it affects daily life.

Imagine one morning in mid-1967, my mom and I arrived at my grandparents' house ready to have a nice visit, playing with my favorite toys, when suddenly I was falling to the floor, bleeding from my mouth, and losing consciousness. Was I dying? Yes I was; it sure felt like it. How would you be in a situation such as this, when you're two years old?

This book is dedicated to all of those who have been affected by epilepsy.

– SK

Introduction

The disease of epilepsy has existed for thousands of years, but only in the past hundred years or so has it begun to be understood. The only symptom of epilepsy is the epileptic seizure and anyone who has experienced or seen such a seizure knows that this experience can be frightening and strange, especially without the knowledge of modern science. Accounts of seizures have been recovered from the first days of recorded history and can even be found in the bible. These records tend to be highly superstitious and religious, though a few of the more scientifically minded have provided more empirical observations. Epilepsy comes from a Greek word meaning "to hold or seize," and people who have epilepsy have seizures. You might also hear a seizure called a convulsion, fit, or spell.

Your brain cells are constantly sending out electrical signals that travel along nerves to the rest of the body. These signals tell the muscles to move so you can do your normal activities. During a seizure, a person's muscles tighten and relax rapidly or stop moving completely. Seizures come on suddenly, and people who have them cannot control their muscles while they are having a seizure.

Depending on where in the brain a seizure is happening, a person's behavior may change in different ways. If too many brain cells are sending signals at the same time, it causes an overload, and a person may pass out and shake all over. People who have epilepsy may have seizures only once in a while or as frequently as every day. Doctors have attempted to explain and cure this strange phenomenon through a wide variety of methods.

The first mention of epilepsy is found with the Babylonians – almost as old as known civilization. They believed it to be caused by the presence of demons, and the different types of seizures depended on the type of demon that inhabited the individual. Though they made observations, there was no mention or development of a cure, even a superstitious one. The Greeks also have records of epilepsy and called it the "Sacred Disease." The Greeks believed that epilepsy was the result of a curse from the gods, delivered for the offense of the goddess Selene. It was believed that if you spent a night in the temple of Selene she would come to you in a dream and tell you how to remove the curse.

In 400 B.C. Hippocrates, the father of medicine, offered another view of epilepsy, that it was just another natural disease and could be treated through natural methods. He supported the use of medicine and control of the diet in order to cure this disease based on his theories of medical methodology. While his methods were hardly scientific he was the first to consider epilepsy to be a natural disorder – and would be the only one to do so for centuries.

After the Greeks, the Romans took a view similar to that of the Babylonians as to the nature of epilepsy. They believed that the disease was also caused by the presence of demons in a person, and that if the person breathed on or touched another, the demon would spread to the other person unless that person spit immediately. In Roman society those who had epilepsy were shunned and isolated, thus setting a precedent for the treatment of epileptics that would last until the enlightenment nearly two thousand years later. Romans also developed a novel and highly pervasive treatment for epilepsy, using the blood of a murdered individual, particularly the blood of a gladiator.

Philosophers suggested other treatments that would be helpful including consuming parts of the human body such as the liver, which made the process of curing the disease a form of cannibalism. This treatment was used for quite a while, with the last known instance as recent as 1908. The introduction of anti-epileptic drugs eventually put an end to the blood-cure.

Throughout the Middle Ages and the Renaissance, epilepsy took on religious connotations again as it did in Greece though there was a difference in opinion between the common people and the nobility as to the nature of the disease. The nobility and the church believed epilepsy not to be a disease at all, but rather a sign of prophetic powers and great intelligence. The common people found it to be a terrible illness and sought a cure for it through contact with holy relics. The Malleus Mallificarum, a guide to witch hunting, provided a third take on seizures by designating them as the sign of witchhood, and many died because of it. This broad social perception of the disease occurred because of both the highly variable nature of the seizures and because of the degree of difference between the classes.

The enlightenment began to change the way epilepsy was looked at, and it was once again believed to be a natural disease. This time the theory was widely accepted. Without the benefit of modern science to allow theories to develop or the ability to research the nature of the brain, epilepsy was still misunderstood. It was believed to be a form of insanity, and considered contagious, resulting in epileptics being confined in mental hospitals away from the other patients. Although the beginnings of dealing with epilepsy as a disease were crude, scientific research into the subject would result in epilepsy being considered in a different light.

Shelley Kobelsky

The first electrical theory of epilepsy was described by Robert Bentley Todd in 1849 in Lumleian lectures he delivered to the Royal College of Physicians. The first person actually credited with the electrical theory was John Hughlings Jackson in 1873. It was held that epilepsy was the result of erratic electrical discharges throughout the entire body, though the brain was not designated as the source at the time. Jackson also recognized that he could not fully explain the sensory alterations with this theory, but left it for future scientists to discover new things and better define his beginning theory of epilepsy as an electrical abnormality.

In the 1930s, the first method for testing the electrical hypothesis for epilepsy was discovered by Hans Berger when he invented the EEG (Electroencephalogram). The eccentric electrical patterns that occurred in the brain during an epileptic seizure proved the problem to indeed be electrical and also showed that its origin was in the brain. Almost ten years later, in 1939, the first animal model for epilepsy was developed allowing the disease to be studied, and treatment methods explored. Also in this year, the first drug to treat epilepsy was developed. After this a variety of drugs were created. Other treatments were developed and refined to create the current range of treatment available for the disease.

Even with the massive strides in changing the way we look at epilepsy, the disease carried with it a strong stigma that would last all the way into the 1990s. Although no longer believed to be possessed, or killed, or put through terrible treatment methods, epileptics still underwent severe prejudice. Throughout the world, including America, epileptics were sterilized or at least prevented from having children, and most companies would refuse to hire an epileptic. The 1990s *Americans with Disabilities Act* covered epileptics and finally prevented them from being discriminated against. Despite the major leaps forward in the study, treatment, and social view of epilepsy, there is much more to be accomplished and researched in dealing with this highly variable and enigmatic disease. In 2000, a massive conference was held by the Epilepsy Foundation of America to begin the pursuit of a complete and total cure for all epileptics.

My motive is to be honest and help others face the challenges, giving them hope and faith, hopefully saving lives and families. It is an open discussion, which is important in getting the truth out. This is a truly unfiltered story which covers the terrain and scope of living with epilepsy on a daily basis. For that reason it has taken a lifetime to write.

My first family doctor actually wrote in my medical history that I was mentally retarded – a fact that I didn't discover until I was in my late teens.

Living with epilepsy is like having earthquakes in your head, hence the name, *My Epi•Center*.

1.

Seizures can cause brain damage, so the more seizures one experiences, the more prone one is to acquiring brain damage. Epilepsy is a hidden, strange central nervous system problem which may have grave and even fatal consequences. It is a grim and debilitating diagnosis and trying to cope and live with this disorder is extremely trying. I endured a lot of ridicule. Epilepsy can be considered either a disease or a disorder; as a disease it has a specific identifiable cause and symptoms. As a disorder it is an unwanted condition that's hard to define or identify its cause. In my case epilepsy is a disease because there is a specific identifiable cause.

More than three million men, women and children in North America (that's about one percent) have epilepsy, and nearly four percent will develop epilepsy at some point in their lives. Epilepsy is more common than multiple sclerosis, Parkinson's disease or autism.

Approximately 70% of those with epilepsy are idiopathic. In other words, they don't know why they are having seizures.

I suffer, not lightly, from right temporal lobe epilepsy with both partial and generalized seizures. I believe this book will help others understand the disorder and show how family and others are affected. I found as a child with epilepsy the trauma of epilepsy made me create a different persona to get through; I was bound and determined to live epilepsy-free. Epilepsy is a disorder you can't buy your way out of!

The temporal lobe is the most common site of focal seizures, and the seizures most often begin in childhood or adolescence.

Auras are a warning that a seizure may soon occur. They had a halo-effect over me. I would feel a weird sensation and I used to say "Mommy, I see stars" so that we could get to a safe place. It felt horrible and scary, and was worse than the seizure itself to me. Even though I was lucky to have this premonition it didn't feel that way. Normally within 30 seconds I would begin to have a convulsion and most were grand mal.

As a teenager in the country I would get auras from looking at the empty fields and vegetation, I would get a bad feeling – almost an upset stomach.

Auras didn't always guarantee an oncoming seizure – but it was better than not having a warning.

Auras include an epigastric sensation, fear and various types of visual, olfactory or auditory experiential phenomena. Cognition may be impaired during a seizure, manifesting itself as confusion, a receptive or expressive dysphasia and ataxia, distraction by an experiential phenomenon or amnesia.

The types of seizures affecting patients with idiopathic generalized epilepsy may include:

Grand Mal seizures

Absence seizures

Myoclonic seizures

Generalized Tonic seizures

Generalized Seizures: Symptoms

(Produced by the entire brain)

Grand Mal or Generalized Tonic – Clonic
Unconscious, convulsions, muscle rigidity

Absence – *Staring spells / brief loss of consciousness*

Myoclonic – *Sporadic (isolated), jerking movements*

Clonic – *Repetitive, jerking movements*

Tonic – *Muscle stiffness, rigidity*

Atonic – *Loss of muscle tone*

More women than men were diagnosed with idiopathic generalized epilepsy in two epilepsy populations. Overall, no gender difference was found in localization-related epilepsy, but localization-related symptomatic epilepsies were more frequent in men, and cryptogenic localization-related epilepsies were more frequent in women. The results suggest a gender susceptibility to the development of specific epilepsy subtypes.

Myoclonic epilepsy is a rare genetic seizure that can be mild and cause brief periods of jerkiness in limited parts of the body, such as the face or trunk, or it may be severe, with grand mal seizures, hearing loss, mental damage, and heart problems. Individuals affected with temporal lobe epilepsy had a similar performance to those age matching controls without cortical damage, as to their sound source direction discrimination hearing mechanism (sound source location), and greater loss in the processing of hearing received information for sounds in sequence and tonal patterns (temporal ordering) discrimination mechanism and the recognition of familiar verbal sounds and non-verbal sounds in dichotic hearing (selective attention).

I wrote this book with the support of most of my family (excluding my father) and friends who want me to share my story. Writing this is pretty hard for me because it brings back many nightmares, but once again I want to get the word out on living with epilepsy and how it affects relationships and lifestyles. This is highly relevant to every living being, as tragedies occur without a moment's notice.

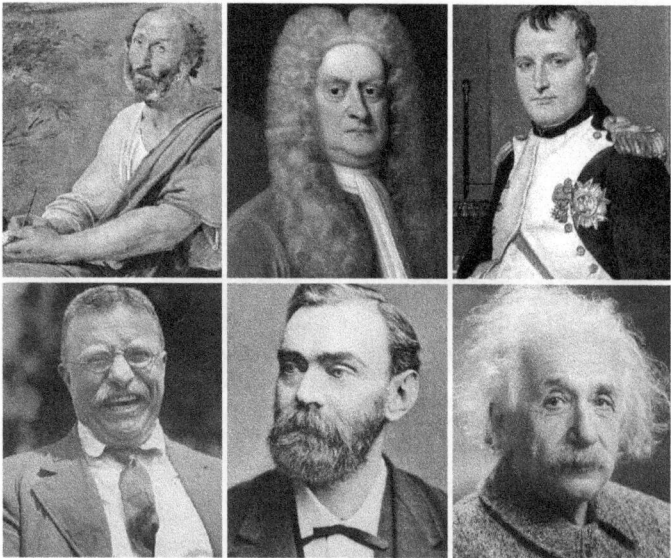

Epilepsy sufferers throughout history, clockwise from top left: Aristotle, Sir Isaac Newton, Napoleon Bonaparte, Albert Einstein, Alfred Nobel and Theodore Roosevelt.

Famous people, both living and throughout history with epilepsy include: Alfred Nobel (who has the same birthday as me, October 21st), Aristotle, Napoleon Bonaparte, Richard Burton, Julius Caesar, Truman Capote, Lewis Carroll, Agatha Christie, Albert Einstein, Danny Glover, Margeaux Hemingway, Mark McAllister (reporter on Global Toronto), Michelangelo, Sir Isaac Newton, Edgar Allen Poe, Pythagoras, Theodore Roosevelt, Vincent Van Gogh, Leonardo da Vinci and Neil Young, to name only a few.*

Many high achievers had epilepsy, which shows that just because you have epilepsy doesn't mean you are incompetent; in fact many suffers have been geniuses. In most cases the cause is unknown.

* *disabled-world.com*

2.

I have two siblings, an older brother and sister and they are part of my story. We were all born within two years and three months. My mother was 17 when she got pregnant with my brother Kevin, the first-born, and my father was 19. My brother was born on my mother's 18th birthday and he seemed healthy and happy.

My sister Sherry was born 11 months after my brother and was perfect at birth, healthy and happy. She seemed to grasp life skills so easily. Soon after her birth we have a picture of her grasping her rattle. Another healthy child; mom was so elated. However, her joy was short-lived as within two to three weeks Sherry began seizing at intervals of time. She would stop breathing, with her arms and legs stiffening, eyes rolled and skin blue.

By the time I was born in October the following year, my mother had been dealing with a sick baby already. Mom was terrified; my dad didn't worry or want to be part of a process which would involve emergencies or doctors, psychiatrists, or the Epilepsy Foundation. My father remained with this attitude all of our lives and continues to do so. He said to me recently that he was not the one that passed the gene on; unbelievable! After all these years, he's never admitted to me that he was the carrier of epilepsy – and his denial hurts. Epilepsy is a closed dialogue in my father's family, not open for discussion for others to find out about, it was considered a demon, not to be shared. Hence a lot of confusion and needless pain continues from this closed dialogue, which reminds me of the song, *King of Pain*. I changed the words to *Queen of Pain*, in my case. I felt the heaviness of the world on my shoulders.

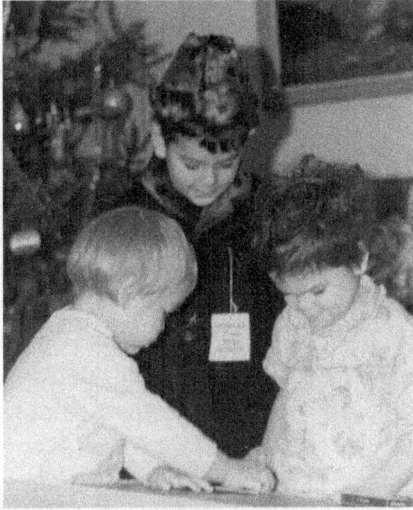

Right: My brother Kevin and sister Sherry (right of picture) with a playmate.

Below: My mother in her thirties.

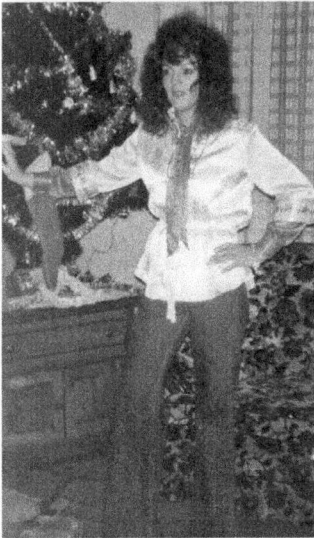

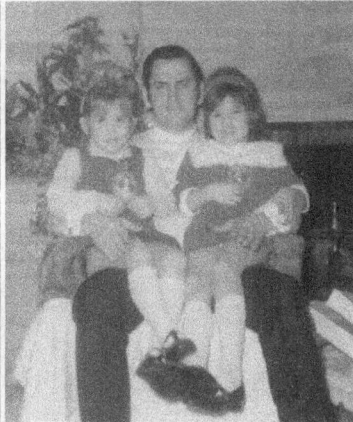

Above: My father with my sister and I when we were very young.

3.

This story is my 9/11 and my goal is just and fair treatment for all afflicted people.

I was born on October 21, 1964 in Windsor, Ontario; a healthy baby with such a promising life ahead; I was never sick. I have a willful nature, am proud and naughty at the same time, yet somehow I was a lovable child in spite of my reckless and demanding personality traits. One couldn't help but notice a quietness about me even though most times I had a lot of excess energy. My mother would say I was an exceptional child. One day, at age two, I was playing in my grandmother's kitchen cupboards with the pots and pans, my favorite toys, and for no apparent reason I suddenly fell on the kitchen floor. My whole body began jerking, I hit my head which caused bleeding and my pupils had rolled back. My first seizure. I lost all consciousness. My mother's family saw me lying there, my four year old brother Kevin standing beside me. He didn't understand what had just happened, which was horrifying for him to see. In order to deal with it I think he went into shock, and from then on he wasn't particularly nice to me.

I recently asked him questions to find out how, and if, he was affected by having two sisters with epilepsy, this is how he responded:

1. How did you adjust (cope) with two siblings with epilepsy?

Didn't have much of a direct effect on me. You were the only one having seizures and they didn't scare me. You were a good sister. Your hyperactivity sometimes drove me around the bend, but no more so than other sisters would have. Sherry never suffered from any symptoms that we were aware of past the time we were young, which I don't remember. The impact of epilepsy was a drop in the bucket compared to our family's instability.

2. How did you cope in school? Did you feel you were being made fun of for having two epileptic sisters?

Never an issue. It (being made fun of) never happened. We moved around a lot and kids hardly knew me, let alone that I had a sister with a medical condition (remember Sherry never showed symptoms at school age). You guys were a couple of years behind me, often at different schools. A non-issue.

3. Did you have a chance to enjoy your childhood?

Absolutely, but there were some really tough times caused by family breakdown and instability.

4. Did you feel obligated to protect Sherry and I from teasing or bullying?

Yes, but, as noted in #2, I can't recall any such incident. You guys got along well with others at school. You were good-natured, nice kids. At times you were hyper, but I never recall that interfering with school or you mentioning being bullied. You were a strong kid. I'd worry more about the other kids making you mad, and you kicking their butt, if I worried at all. But I never did.

5. Did you feel like a surrogate parent, being approached for information or support?

A couple of times, yes, but that was much later, in high school, when Dad was having trouble with the two of you. You guys got kicked around. We had lived with Mom for years, but then Mom decided you should live with Grandma, and Sherry with Dad (at different times). You guys didn't come to me for support because we didn't live together at that time. But there were just a couple of times I stepped in. So not really a surrogate parent providing ongoing support, but a surrogate adult who stepped in if things got out of hand.

6. When you were under the age of 12 did you have fear of Sherry or I having a seizure? Did you know what to do? Did it cause you extra stress? Were you afraid of one of us dying?

No. You'd had hundreds of them and come out fine. It was normal. I'd just let you chill out until you were done. Sherry never had seizures at an age where I was old enough to remember them (she was done with them before I was 7 - when we lived on Huron Line) so a non-issue for her. Again, overall, the direct effects of the epilepsy on me were quite small. Aside from being hyper (today they call it ADHD), you guys were nice kids, and fun. Great attitudes. Liked to learn. So for me the family story is not about epilepsy, but the breakup and subsequent moving around.

Everyone was traumatized, they didn't know what or why this happened. Everyone was crying and terrified, my grandmother will never forget this day, in her home, in front of her eyes. My uncle Ray, who was 18, called 911. My mother tried comforting me, she was so scared that I might die so she thought she was trying to save me. The seizure felt like it lasted forever. A minute later I began seizing again, so my uncle Ray took us to the hospital. In Windsor in those days an ambulance wasn't necessarily dispatched even for a baby in distress. Uncle Ray drove my mother and me to the Emergency Room. An ambulance would have felt safer for us all. By the time we got there I had stopped seizing. In the ER, the doctors were checking if the symptoms could be due to parental abuse, they interviewed my mother, took blood tests, x-rays, and nothing worked. This ritual was repeated many times. Gradually these episodes, not yet labelled epilepsy, were taking their toll on my health. The dream of being a healthy girl was over. It was like I had died (the healthy me) and a different person was born (a child with seizures). In losing that perfect child I became a poster child for finding a cure for these seizures/fits, whatever they were. I got pity — which didn't work, so then I got frustrated, feeling responsible for the sadness — a heavy load for a child to carry. I was brought up with depression and fear and flight. That's how my life changed completely.

My mom and my Aunt Lynn would take us on outings daily, hoping somehow, in spite of the fear of seizures, that my sister and I would experience childhood joys. My mother was an energetic 20 year-old when I was born, her last child. I can't recall my sister's bouts with episodes, however I can recall the safety net of a large loving extended family on both sides. My mother's family was not only helpful, they were deeply involved in creating my personality and character of today. I will give insight to these precious memories as I write about my journey with epilepsy. I'd like to quote Alfred Nobel who stated "It will be brief and concise, which is eloquent."

My parents divorced when I was seven years old. Pictures of me having a seizure couldn't be found as no one wanted to see me having a seizure let alone take pictures.

My question is this: "Have you ever seen anybody having a seizure? Were you afraid? How did you handle it?" Within those crucial first years after age two, I was hurt so much emotionally, physically and relationally. We as a family cracked, broke.

We were to learn how much power epilepsy carries; it can ruin lives.

It's been a real challenge trying to be normal. I look

normal until you see me fall on the ground or fall over on the chair. My maternal grandmother, who is an inspiration to me, was hit by a streetcar when she was three years old in the mid-1920s and was in a coma for a few weeks. The resident doctor gave her up for dead, there was no neuro-surgery back then.

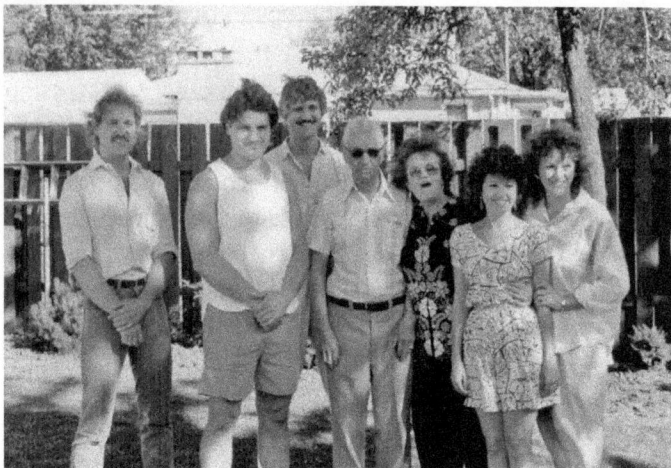

My maternal grandparents and their five children. From left to right: My uncle Don, uncle Ray, uncle Ron, grandpa Rene Gauthier, grandma Genevieve Gauthier, aunt Lynn and my mother Joyce.

A new graduate doctor came on staff and tried a new technique; it was one of the first brain operations. The doctor cut open her scalp, removed the damaged area and soaked it in alcohol washing her brain and then he sewed her scalp back together. She woke up in an isolation unit and wasn't allowed to move her head. She wasn't allowed visits from her mother as this would prove to be too much for this primitive surgery. However, her dad was allowed to bring her ice cream once a day. She is now 94 years old and it's a wonder she is still alive. She always had to be so careful not to hit her head as it could have killed her. Somehow she became intuitively aware of danger – to this day she is like a prize fighter – always coming out of any negative situation a winner.

4.

Doctors tried various medical interventions on me, but nothing worked; the medicine caused side effects such as slurred speech (cruelly referred to as "talking like a retarded person" in the 1960s), balance problems and dizziness. I was unable to go on rides that spun because I would get all dizzy and sick. Also, my bone density was compromised which caused brittle bones (later as an adult I broke my right femur in a fall; another nightmare). Today when I talk, my speech seems monotone except when I am telling jokes. I feel many people treat me differently, as if I'm intellectually challenged. Having epilepsy has shaped my personality and affected my self esteem. I am not comfortable speaking in groups. I hear my speech as slow and I believe I see myself as others see me, but I know differently. My spirit is strong, I feel what drove me to keep moving forward was my faith in God and my grandmother's story as well as having a very close relationship with her. Since my father and uncle grew out of their seizures, I felt they were lucky – if you believe in luck!

Eventually my seizures became more erratic and I needed to go to *The Hospital for Sick Children* in Toronto, a four hour drive. I was seizing all the way (*status epilepticus* or constant seizures). My life was at stake but my father decided to work instead of taking time off. My uncle Ross and Aunt Lynn offered to take time off work (he was a police officer) so he drove my mother and me to the hospital driving well over the speed limit. Half way there he was stopped by a provincial police officer on the highway. He showed his police badge, explaining to the officer why he was speeding, but the officer gave him a $200 ticket anyway. Again, there should have been paramedics or a helicopter. In spite of this we made it alive, barely. The doctors said I should have been dead, my blood sugar was so low. I was the first person with such a low blood sugar level to survive, setting a record.

At the hospital, convulsing often caused a lot of unnecessary damage and hurt, yet somehow at times I could still have fun. I had fun sharing my food with other kids.

I was a little ham and social butterfly, the nursing staff found me to be personable, adorable. They felt my mom could go home, I seemed to settle right in with the other kids, but my mom struggled with leaving. After her departure I would act out, beating up the kids, throwing my food at them instead of sharing it. My behavior changed completely and this would lead to a seizure. I screamed and was writhing in pain. I was tied to a bed in the hospital after my mother was sent home, the nurses thought I might be a danger to myself or others. During this time in hospital my brother stayed with his paternal grandparents and my sister with my maternal grandparents; my mother had to stay in the hospital with me to avoid more seizures and damage. In those days there was no support or counselling; there wasn't a Ronald McDonald house to assist challenged families. My mother had to pay for her food and lodging so she could be with me at the hospital. It was a divided system, families were not together as one parent needed to be at the hospital with the sick child and the other at home working and taking care of the other children, if they had more than one. Now, when I think of the lack of support, care, and love for me, my sister, brother and mother, I'm overwhelmed with the survival instincts that are inherent in my family.

Upon my mother's return I stopped convulsing and once again the doctors couldn't find anything. My stress escalated to a dangerous level whenever my mother was taken from me. Anything stressful, emotional or physical, could trigger an attack. I would often have an aura, a sensation about 30 seconds before a seizure, so this would give me a bit of time to get to a safe place. My mother would ask before going on a ride at the carnival if I felt I would be okay. She would say "Are you sure?" I'd answer "Yes, yes, I'm okay." She trusted me and then allowed me to go on rides.

The truth of the matter is that you can no more win a war than you can win a seizure, they both involve explosions in your head.

Still, we never gave up, I was later admitted to Hotel Dieu Hospital in my hometown of Windsor. I wasn't allowed to eat anything with Lutein, all I could eat was bananas and goat's milk for two to three weeks; just long enough to determine that Lutein wasn't the cause. It felt like torture. Especially at Easter when the other children got chocolate eggs from the Easter Bunny. I got what looked like a chocolate egg but turned out to be a plastic egg filled with bananas. I knew instantly it wasn't a chocolate egg. I threw it across the room and refused to eat it, which broke my mother's heart. I knew I wasn't supposed to have chocolate, but when my mother left I talked another mother into sharing *Smarties* from the Easter Bunny which I smothered all over my face. I was so happy. One unhappy doctor put a "DO NOT FEED" sign on my bed and all the tests had be run again. Of course, Lutein wasn't the cause. To this day I still don't really like to eat bananas. Doctors suggested putting a spoon in my mouth, under my tongue, so I wouldn't choke or swallow my tongue. Another old wives tale was putting a teaspoon of honey in my mouth which didn't help. There were a few other attempts – all were doomed to failure. Like my paternal grandmother giving us some herbs from her hometown in Saskatchewan that were supposed to cure what ailed me (seizure disorder).

Between two and four years old I would get viruses and bacteria from the hospital and had many high fevers. I had fevers to 106 degrees and the doctors ordered my mother to quickly immerse my body in a bathtub full of ice water to bring my temperature down, as there was not time for the hospital. My mother and I were both moaning and crying as she held me safely in her arms while I was seizing. Sounds cruel, doesn't it?

5.

I began to be hyperactive – the really bad type, nowadays called ADHD. Many people wonder what came first, epilepsy or ADHD (hyperactivity). Like what came first, the chicken or the egg? From experience and research I've discovered epilepsy causes hyperactivity. It could be from the medication, or from the part of the brain the epilepsy affects. Prior to seizures I was not hyper, I was good-natured.

Some advice for families and friends of people suffering from epilepsy: "Embrace the person as if they were healthy." The top concern should be to ask what is needed: ...a hug ...lay down?

I feel that it's the parents' responsibilities to give their children dignity and kindness no matter what the situation entails. The response varies with the type of seizure. Since I had auras mine were fear-based; my mother would hold and rock me and I could intuitively feel this. As a young child with epilepsy I had developed a strong intuition. I seemed to know who to reach out to and knew who was there for me.

I could either stay in this aura or allow it to pass and move on, even with a headache. During these auras I would think to myself "I'll be okay." I would be in the fight or flight mode (survival mode trying to stop the transmission from the aura to a seizure). This worked once in a while. I

internalized this coping mechanism hoping to beat the seizures. The alternative flight would be to just let the seizure
occur, losing consciousness and losing control, a horrible
choice. Also, I knew I was different and felt loved less than
I felt before having seizures.

I became highly perceptive from having epilepsy,
and I have a heightened sense of smell. I feel that I occasionally react inappropriately to constructive criticism and
feel unjustly judged because I am not healthy.

My mother had to put bars (high side-bars) around
my crib so I couldn't climb out. However, being me, I found
a way out. On hearing the bell from the ice-cream truck
I jumped out of the bedroom window onto our crushed
stone driveway. I was crying and the neighbour heard me
yelling for ice cream. I was not in my bed as my mother
thought. The driver was yelling at me, not knowing what
to do, as I was hanging on the back of his ice cream truck!
I could have fallen off, had a seizure and died. All I could
think of was the ice cream! I felt I could do anything and
nothing would stop me, no pain or anything. This was quite
scary for my parents, mom looked at hands torn from the
crushed stone but I didn't cry. They never knew what form
of escape I would try next. Sometimes, just to be defiant,
when I was about to get into trouble, if the stove was hot,
I'd put my hand on the element and say "see, that doesn't
hurt." It was a way of saying "There's no point in punishing
me as it won't hurt anyway." This ADHD had given me su-
perpowers.

I was two years old when my brother Kevin, at the
age of four, split his head open. My grandparents had hired
a contractor to build their new house and my brother was
playing on a dirt pile nearby and fell down a 13 foot embankment and split his head on the cement footing. My
uncle Ray jumped down the embankment, picked up Kevin
and came running with Kevin in his arms with a shocked

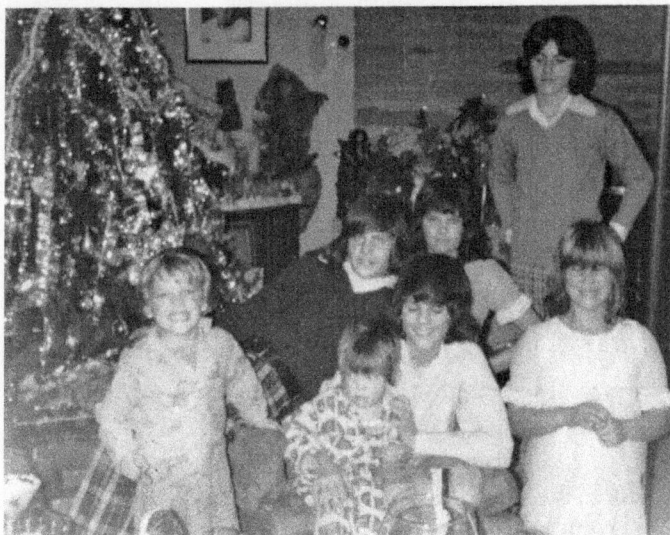

Christmas at my maternal grandparents house. From left to right: Cousin Todd, brother Kevin holding cousin Shawn, stepbrother Jimmy, sister Sherry, stepbrother Steven and me at the front right side of photo.

expression on his face. All my mother and her family could see were Kevin's bloody handprints on Ray's t-shirt. Uncle Ray was in shock. This happened on the same day as Sherry, my sister was diagnosed by our family doctor as mentally retarded.

When I was three years old we went to the London Psychiatric Institute, a last resort for diagnosis. While I was there I got impetigo, a contagious bacterial infection most common among preschool children, which causes red sores that can break open, ooze fluid, and develop a yellow-brown crust. I also got boils all over my legs, arms and genitals. I screamed as my mother was breaking them, cleaning out wounds and cutting off my long golden curls. She cried seeing me hurt so badly. The doctors and nurses were still unable to stop me from convulsing; they couldn't figure out the cause of my seizures.

As a result of these convulsions I had many hospital stays, and my family doctor wanted to keep me home, away from the sick people in the hospital. A nice thought but impossible with my severe case. I was a friendly little girl and made many friends in the hospital, even with a little boy with just one ear and a disfigured face who everyone else was avoiding.

Finally, when I was about four years old, relatives from out west came to our house visiting and saw my sister and I convulsing. They told my mother that this disorder was genetic, as my paternal grandmother had seizures and my father and his identical twin brother had seizures as well. My paternal aunt died when she was just one month old in a seizure. Both my father and uncle grew out of their seizures by their late-teens, but not without their own pain and suffering caused by others. When my mother found out about the epilepsy, although they didn't call it that, she was shocked and could finally put all the pieces together about what was happening to her children. My sister and I – two out of three of my father's children – had epilepsy. None of my paternal cousins had the disorder, but they are carriers.

6.

My epilepsy is definitely genetic, as my nephew Matthew got it as a child and my cousin's daughter (on my father's side of the family) got epilepsy as well. I feel my mission is to break the cycle of epilepsy and open the closet doors with open dialogue so that others won't have to go through unnecessary pain and they can deal with epilepsy. They can treat it early and give the person a relatively normal life. This is why it is so important to be honest and share open dialogue with others; in order to manage the disorder without any unnecessary damage. As children, my father and uncle (identical twins) would walk a long way to school and the teachers would get so mad at my dad and uncle for having a seizure in class that they would ban them from eating their lunch which would in effect cause more seizures. My father and uncle would watch each other having seizures and help each other; going to school was like torture, but they had to go no matter what. This is a feeling I understand well; others can be hurtful.

I was labelled as a person with epilepsy (stigmatized) and felt like a misfit; an alien, not part of the world.

For no reason I would suddenly get aggressive and my pupils would dilate. I would have an attack and then feel tired and wanting to sleep afterwards. I was only two years old, yet I knew I was different, there was less joy and laughter. I wasn't the perfect daughter, niece and grandchild.

I would go on rides at the fair and play the games for prizes and have seizures with little warning, if at all. While playing a game at a fair, throwing a dart to hit the bullseye to win a big prize, I felt a seizure coming on, but I was determined to go on, I had a grand mal seizure right after throwing the dart. I somehow managed to hit the bullseye, winning a big stuffed animal which I was so proud of. Others were yelling at my mother to call 911, so she would then try to calm them down, explaining that I was having a seizure and to give me some space; that I would come out of it. This worked, calming people down.

Sometimes I would have an aura that was not followed by a seizure, so I never really knew when I was going to have a seizure. The aura was a horrible feeling and mom would ask, "What is it you are feeling?" I would tremble in fear and cry out, "The sky is falling, the sky is falling!" My paternal grandfather put me down his kitchen chute and used a fan belt on me if he thought I wasn't listening to him. He was from a poor family and when we ate if I couldn't finish my meal he'd punish me badly, including as I mentioned, the fan belt. I learned to beat him at his own game later and would go to washroom right after eating and barf in the toilet to let out the food that I couldn't eat; it wasn't a nice visit when we went over there. Another time he locked me outside in his garage alone, it felt like forever, this is not my imagination. He punished me for my behaviour which was often prior to a seizure. I felt he was awfully mean to me. I remember having a seizure in the garage, laying on the floor and waking up alone, scared. I didn't know how long he was going to leave me in there for.

On another occasion I remember scratching the neighbour's brand new car on one side. I was playing with their granddaughter, Lorna, and then I jumped the fence, scratched the car, and came home before having a seizure. I was upset about something. The neighbour was really upset as well, and said I was the only child she has ever hated.

It is strange how an earthquake in your head seems less of a catastrophe than the first scratch on your new car.

At a research hospital in London, doctors were trying to find out why I was hyper yet my sister was so quiet and introverted. My sister and I were on separate floors, there was a floor for hyper children and another for introverted children. I always wanted my mother with me, if she went away I wouldn't eat my food. The nurses didn't like me for this reason.

As a little girl at the fair I sometimes said "Mommy, I see stars."

She knew what that meant. I may have a seizure. Living with this was like an epi-center in my head, knowing the explosion could go off at any moment. My mother would always say "Jesus Loves You" and "I love you" during my seizures, hoping I was hearing this and hoping I wouldn't die from the seizure. I used to try to think of something else and hope to distract myself from having a seizure. Sometimes this worked. My mother would call me "Miss Epi" since I had a severe seizure disorder, trying to make light of the situation. Humour in many forms is a pacifier.

We had a little dog for a while but had to give it away because it was so sensitive and empathetic; when I had a seizure, it would convulse, so it was terribly unhealthy for the dog. My mother had to give the dog away for its own health. In retrospect, with proper training, he would have been a great service dog. Also, watching my sister have seizures was hard on me, sometimes it would cause me to have a seizure. My sister didn't have auras, she would stare and lose consciousness for a moment. She grew out of these *Absence* seizures at around seven, but that's another story. Hers was due to frontal lobe epilepsy.

In the winter when it was sunny, with snow on the ground, I would walk to the mall, about 1.5 km from home. Even with sunglasses on, the strong reflection caused me to have a grand mal seizure, so I fell in the snow and woke up a few minutes later with a bad headache, but kept walking hoping I wouldn't have another fit. Simple things like taking a bath, walking, shopping, swimming and using stairs leave people with epilepsy vulnerable. Even after recovering from the seizure they may end up with brain damage or mental retardation.

Living with epilepsy meant I should have lived in a calm, stable home. Instead, epilepsy was the reason I wasn't living this way.

Shelley Kobelsky

7.

As children, my two siblings and I moved around often. I lived in many places between Windsor and Toronto in Southern Ontario. Moving around like this from my father's to my mother's was incredibly hard on me, I know it caused many seizures. I could seizure anytime, but any excitement, good or bad, would often cause more seizures. On holidays, we would go to my maternal grandparents for Christmas Eve until all hours in the morning and celebrate, have a lot of fun and then go to my paternal grandparents on Christmas Day. I would get so excited to go to my grandparents, having fun on Christmas Eve and Christmas Day, I would end up having seizures. Many people around would get scared that I might not come out of the seizure. I'd just go to bed and want to sleep, later waking up with a massive headache. Special occasions and holidays always came with a bad cost (seizures), but I always had hope that they would go away and never return. I lived with them for 20 years pretty constantly. I would try to keep calm during adversity and good times to avoid setting off another seizure. I found what got me through was the fun I had at my maternal grandparents with my aunt, uncles, and grandparents. We would go to the trailer on the lake and have marshmallows on the fire pit and fish. I loved that. Also, my uncles had many friends which were like uncles to me and I got to play cards and pinball with them, it was great, no stress. They were a vital part of my survival.

A major coping mechanism for me was music, I would listen, figure out all the words and sign along. I still love music, it seems to have a calming effect on me, and I would try to distract an oncoming seizure with a song in my head which would stop the transmission and seizures occasionally. One of my theme songs is *American Pie*, the part that says "the day the music died" which is like my first seizure was the day my healthy self-died. Another song is *Live Like You Were Dying* by Tim McGraw; this song was about family and friends with cancer; people with limited time which gave them a new perspective on life (live life to the fullest becoming the best person you can).

When I went into grade one, I couldn't sit for more than 30 seconds at a time so the teachers would put me back and forth from the regular to the special (slow) class. I wasn't retarded, so they put me back in the regular class, teachers didn't know what class to put me in; they thought I was hyperactive. In those days there were no ADHD labels like today and I think my hyperactivity was a side effect of my medicine. When I was about six years old my father and uncle stole us from school and my mother knew nothing about this. Her lawyer never thought my father could do this. My father wanted his children living with him, even though he wasn't home much. In court he said he wanted his children going to the same school until the divorce was through. The judge said he didn't want to hear from my dad, and my mother got custody. Getting a court date took two years. In those days, women and children had no rights. Nowadays, custody battles are done right away, before divorce, for the children's sake. My mother had a lot of support; my grandparents, aunt and uncles who were always there for me. My mother's attorney, a prominent lawyer in Windsor, told her that there was no need to be concerned over custody, it was automatically hers. My father had a lawyer as well, he applied to a Higher Court unbeknownst to my mom or her lawyer. In court, I remember the judge asking who I wanted to live with, and I said, "My mother." We ended up living with my father and had two different Jamaican maids, one at a time, live with us. It was 100 degrees outside and I remember the maid turning the heat on, this also caused more seizures. I would ask my father when he got home if I could turn the air conditioning on and he'd say no, he would only allow a fan blowing really hot air around. I therefore couldn't sleep as it was too hot! Finally, two years later, the Higher Court gave my mother full custody with my dad having visiting rights every three weeks for a weekend but we rarely wanted to go. The following year we moved again.

We also moved often because my seizures scared the neighbours, they didn't know what to do and were afraid to invite me over in case I had a seizure and died. However, I was lucky that my mother wasn't over-protective and allowed me to live relatively normally, so I got to do things many people suffering from epilepsy don't get to. I was allowed to swim, go boating, and go to fairs amongst many other fun things. There were some relatives that I felt didn't treat me right; my aunt (father's sister-in-law), didn't want me sitting on her couch in case I had a seizure and blood came out of my mouth, it was a dreadful existence. However, for my sister and me existing was not an option, as we'd rather live and endure the pain rather than just survive.

Sometimes I would make a joke in my head to get through this horrible existence. I would think to myself, "Oops, my brain just hit a bad area, it farted."

My mother tried having a normal life with two of three children being disabled. There was no help in those days, we were alone left to deal with all the problems, and we were pioneers. I am a pioneer for having my brain surgery in the early stages of this treatment. In order to achieve a better lifestyle and to make it easier for others, our family got the ball rolling in many different facets as explained. It was hard to be a pioneer, undergoing testing with no solutions in sight, blindly; but I believed something could be found and I forged ahead! In order to achieve a better lifestyle and make it easier for others, I had the determination of a winner, not a whiner.

Later when I was about eight years old my mother met a fellow at her workplace who she fell in love with. He was from Oakville, Ontario, and a few months later my family was introduced to his. He had three children and we seemed to like each other. A month later, we moved to Oakville with my mother's boyfriend and his three children.

We were like the Brady Bunch, in this case the Phillips bunch. We seemed to get along like one big happy family. I got along well with my two stepbrothers and one stepsister, whom I'm still in contact with. Living with three new siblings, as fun as it was, was hard on me as my mother wasn't as attentive to me and I could feel it which inevitably caused seizures. I was in grade three when we lived in Oakville and I knew I was smart, my teacher wanted to skip me to grade four, but since my sister was in that class they didn't want siblings in the same class, I was held back. I excelled in spelling and math. I am an over-achiever, I have always had to compensate for my illness trying to fit in and be normal. I had a crush on the boy next door, he was about three years older than me and we slept in the tent together. Of course my mother thought we were playing inside.

8.

After my parents separated they made an arrangement whereby my father would take us on a trip every year somewhere during shutdown at the plant he worked at. We saw many places, I remember my first helicopter ride over the Smoky Mountains in Tennessee – what a beautiful sight! We also drove to Washington, DC, New York City, Pittsburgh and Virginia. We went to the top of the Empire State Building and called my mother for her birthday and years later my mother called my brother from the top of the CN Tower when it opened for his birthday; they share the same birthday, both on August 9th.

As for school, I excelled, but was the recipient of many mean jokes, people making fun of me during and after a seizure. My favorite subjects were math and spelling. I always felt like classmates were treating me as if I was slow, but if anything I needed a class for really smart people, not a special class for children with learning disabilities. In grade four in Windsor I was doing the grade eight spelling book, finished it, and the teacher put me back to grade four spelling. I lived with my mom's parents (grandparents) for a year and had a great year, their home was stable and they treated me like gold, so I barely had any seizures. Once before a seizure I was mad and I scratched my grandfather's back, he was so kind-hearted and I didn't get punished for hurting him. I used to get up in the morning, my grandfather would make us breakfast (bacon & eggs) and he would tell me to go swimming while he was cooking breakfast, then call me in when it was ready. We would drive to one of his construction sites, look at the property, and then return home and I would get ready and go to school. My grandmother would sew me dresses and drive me around to different relatives, to weddings and different places, it was a lot of fun.

I swam in my grandparent's outdoor pool, particularly in the summer. My grandfather used to throw coins at the bottom of the pool and all the grandchildren would race to the bottom to get the money. I almost always won the race as I was a fast swimmer; people would call me "fish" and "sea dog" because I loved swimming so much.

I actually believe that I could have been an Olympic swimmer, but once again epilepsy held me back. Life felt so unfair, but I kept trying to tolerate living with epilepsy, plugging away daily. I managed to make friends with the next door neighbour and we had a lot of fun together. We camped, swam, played games. I got to live like a normal person for a while. Christmas Eve was at my maternal grandparents' home pretty well every year and we had such good times. My uncle's group of best friends would come over, we'd play games and stay up all night. We had a feast after going to Midnight Mass and then open our presents, there were so many under the tree. This was a highlight for me, it helped me get through the daily struggles knowing I could have a lot of fun.

However, in grade five, I moved to the Niagara region with my mother and step-siblings and began having more seizures. All the moving and commotion, including living with three other children, was hard on me. We stayed there for two years where I saw doctors but none of them could control my seizures.

Day after day I would try to get through without

people at school laughing and making fun of me. Children can be absolutely cruel if you're different. I was always considered a nice person, but weird, so many people would shun me like the plague. It was lonely and frustrating. I would usually sit at the back of the room so that most people wouldn't notice me.

One weekend I decided to try something.

We lived near the Welland Canal which has lift bridges that open and close for ships to get through the St. Lawrence Seaway. I decided to get on the lift bridge while it was going up. About half way up the conductor saw me and announced over the public address system that I was to get off, but I didn't, so he stopped the bridge. A minute later, I jumped off. I could have easily had a seizure, fallen into the canal and died. My mother and stepfather didn't know I had done this and luckily when I jumped off I didn't hit the side, fall in the canal and die.

The point is I tried to experience life in spite of my condition. I had many seizures and life is unusually tough, I felt like giving up many times as my case was so gruelling. However, I believed maybe at 16 I would grow out of my seizures like my uncle and father did in their late-teens. My father used to take us on Sunday drives and I would get motion sickness. It was worse when I sat in the back seat, and driving out to the country. The view often caused me to have seizures, so I hated drives through the countryside, I lost consciousness and woke up with a severe headache feeling like I was in a fog.

In grade six we moved again, this time to Burlington with my mom, where I had to meet all new teachers and make new friends again. However, we managed to find a doctor that I thought was excellent! I was still convulsing often, and again many people were afraid of me, not knowing what to expect or when to expect it.

I tried to get through another year hoping some-thing would work out with my health, but again nothing worked!

9.

I went to the Epilepsy Foundation in Toronto feeling hopeful that they could help me, that they could understand my problem. Again, I was disappointed, they weren't helpful, and they didn't know what they were talking about, giving wrong advice most of the time. In grade eight, I moved back to Windsor and finished up going to three different schools. My father moved into a different house across the city since his girlfriend didn't want to live on the outskirts where there were no buses.

When I moved back to Windsor in grade eight, my father was still living on the outskirts of the city on a busy highway, so I took a bus to school. I got so bored out there, there wasn't much to do, you needed a car to go places and I was too young. I lasted four months, then I decided to move into the city with my grandparents where everything was close and safe. I stayed there three months and after my father moved into his new house, in the city, with his girlfriend and her three children, I moved back with him, to give my grandparents a break while I finished grade eight – not that they complained!

With all the moving during grade eight, I ended up missing an important function: my confirmation, because every school held this at a different time. Confirmation is a Roman Catholic rite of passage and I was so disappointed to miss it.

My brother used to drive my sister and me to visit my mother in Oakville, almost a four hour drive. We would quiz each other in the car about music trivia and that's probably why I know the words to so many songs. It was a good idea, it kept us busy in the car. Also, with my father we used to say all the US states in order, he'd see if we could remember them all and it made a game to help make the car rides fun. I remember going to have a blood test and I had to fast for twelve hours before. After the appointment crossing the main street in Windsor I had a seizure in the middle of the busy street because my glucose was so low. I went to Wendy's for some lunch and took the bus home, tired and with a bad headache.

My father's girlfriend had two boys and a girl. I got along surprisingly well with her and her youngest son; not her older son and daughter. I had many grand mal and petit mal seizures due to the conflict and instability in the house. Most of the time I took care of the youngest child. I would take him on the bus with me – he was ten years younger than me.

They stayed for almost two years, then my father's girlfriend and children moved out, so my father, brother, sister and I lived together. My sister and I would do all the cooking and cleaning at home, including cutting the lawn; I was still convulsing frequently, pretty much daily.

10.

I went to a private high school from grade 9 to part of grade 11, the same school my brother and parents went to. Many people didn't want to talk to me, they were snobby, and I was abnormal (misfit).

I'll give my father credit for helping me once in grade 10 with my homework, explaining the principle. Then I aced the subject.

I worked part-time at a fast food restaurant, I was hired to do drinks. One day at work I worked in the fries department and I had a seizure. I almost fell into the hot grease but luckily for me someone caught me or I am sure I would have been badly burned. They fired me since it was not safe for me to work.

At the time, my mother and her boyfriend lived near Ottawa and I decided to go canoeing on the river with my two cousins. My mother had shown my cousins what to do in case I had a seizure in the middle of the river. My cousins were about ten years old, and certainly smart and caring. They listened to my mother's instructions, so when I later had a seizure they knew exactly what to do, and managed to get us back to land safely. My cousins are like brothers to me and they were never afraid, they would do anything for me. They didn't judge me or make me feel different and ended up being more compassionate to others.

My aunt developed ovarian cancer at 28 years old and she, her husband and children moved next door. In spite of having seizures, I babysat my cousins, they seemed to treat me normally and we helped each other as needed. Watching me have seizures must have affected them, but perhaps in a positive way, as they were more compassionate and caring to the issues of other people.

In grade 11 I moved to Mississauga with my mother and new stepfather Andy for eight months, and while living there I had a grand mal seizure right in the middle of downtown! Cars slammed their brakes on. I ended up in an ambulance and had to stay in the hospital until I came out of the seizure. It was a wonder I wasn't killed!

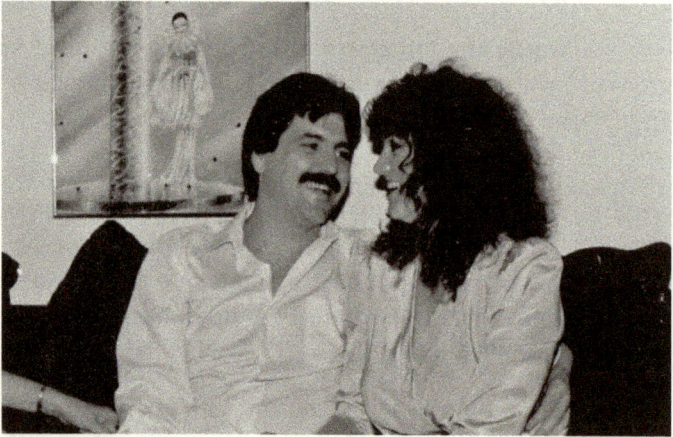

My mother Joyce Gauthier and stepfather Andy Brown

My mother and stepfather moved to Calgary a few months later so I moved back to my father's in Windsor while I was in grade 12. I later got another part-time job in a car wash, wiping down the inside and outside of cars, and earned three dollars per hour plus tips. I was trying to save up to go on my first big plane ride with my sister to Calgary to visit my mom. I managed to accomplish my goal, and it was such a beautiful place that I wanted to stay there.

In Calgary, I went to the Epilepsy Foundation. The counsellor was great, she had suffered from epilepsy years before, but she seemed normal. She had great advice and knew what she was talking about, and by sharing her experience and knowledge she gave me hope again. I was tested and told that I should be an investigator, accountant, politician or lawyer. At that time in Calgary you could go to university after grade 12, you didn't need grade 13 like in Ontario; I wanted to moved there but my mother wasn't sure how long they were going to stay since her family was in Ontario, so I ended up moving back to Ontario with my father.

Whenever I was living with my father, he always wanted me working, making some money no matter what! In grade 13 he got me a good part-time job at Chrysler as a TPT (Temporary part-time); it paid well. I worked in the big van plant on the gate line.

Once, while at work, I got excited because my sister, who lived in London, was coming to visit, so with only 15 minutes left on my shift I had a grand mal seizure. Before convulsing I remember saying to my co-workers, "Hey guys, I have to sit down for a few minutes." I was having an aura. I ended up having a grand mal seizure and was in the hospital from about midnight to 2:00 am. A co-worker stayed with me for a couple hours. I think since I had told the guys I had to sit down and then had a seizure in a safe spot I didn't get fired. Chrysler then had me checking the electrical and working in the office in the plant.

Also, in grade 13 I wanted a certain mark in biology to graduate with honours. During the final exam I had a grand mal seizure and the teacher told me to go home, but I wanted to get a certain mark so I stayed with a bad headache, managed to finish the exam, and got the mark I wanted. I finished high school and graduated with honours, in spite of my epilepsy and seizures.

11.

The unique issues for women with epilepsy revolve around hormonal changes, including contraception and pregnancy. For example, care of a woman during the child-bearing years – and especially pregnancy – needs special attention to treatment choices and other health concerns, including safety and parenting as well as many other aspects of daily life.

My hormone levels were so low that I didn't experience normal periods. In fact I took medicine to try to get periods but I never had normal ones; once in a while I'd just have some bleeding. I missed out on the *Menarche*, the celebration of a woman's first menstrual cycle. I didn't get the chance to be a young lady with all the feelings that come with falling in love and getting married. I missed out because my ovaries never developed, so this cycle of life never occurred for me and as far as I'm concerned that strengthened my resilience.

My mission has always been to not carry the epilepsy cycle to the next generation, so I did not want to have children. I know I couldn't handle more than one child for an extended period of time. Once, in the late 1980s, I went to a birthday party at work in Toronto; there were many children in a play area like an arena, riding their bikes in circles. I got quite dizzy from watching and hearing all the screaming, so I told my two best friends that I had to step out for 15 minutes, otherwise I might not be able to drive us home. At the time I was the only person with my driver's license so I had to be careful. I took a break then went back 15 minutes later and was feeling fine. We stayed for another hour and then I drove home. This taught me that even though I am great with kids and they love me, I am not healthy enough to take care of children around the clock.

I was unable to attend my prom because of my epilepsy. It seemed like nobody wanted to take me – I am abnormal after all – and teenagers aren't compassionate. Once again I felt like a misfit.

My morals and beliefs didn't allow me to have intercourse before marriage, and I was not going to have children, because I was determined not to pass on the epilepsy gene to the next generation. However, I wondered about having intercourse. I thought maybe if I had an orgasm I would have a seizure, which does happen. This was just another reason why I felt I couldn't have intimate sex with my partner. My sex drive was below average, probably from my medicine, and I always stuck to my belief system at any cost. Medical studies say 95% of seizures occurred after intercourse. Like my work, I would go to any lengths trying to be normal while living in an abnormal body.

By this time any hope that my seizures would stop had vanished, and it seemed living with epilepsy would be forever.

Having these recurring earthquakes in my head is just horrendous. To be safe I would try to sit down when I felt an aura coming on, but seizures were, and are, extremely hard to predict.

12.

I wanted my driver's license so badly but wasn't supposed to drive, because my seizures weren't controlled.

The loss or suspension of a driving license significantly disrupts life, but the medical, emotional and legal impacts of a medically related driving injury to others or to one's self potentially causes greater anguish. I took driving classes and would say prayers in my head hoping to keep myself from having a seizure; it seemed to work. I passed the course and got my license on my first attempt. During the driving test I was once again praying a lot, hoping I wouldn't have a seizure.

A year later I was driving my father's car coming back from my paternal grandparent's house and I felt an aura coming on. I was on a secondary highway near a major highway. I pulled over, a seizure had started and I ended up in the ditch. When the owners of a nearby farmhouse came out to see what had happened, I told them I was just trying to avoid an accident and ended up in the ditch. I was out of the seizure by the time the people came, so I just drove home and luckily nothing happened. I never bought a car until after I had the seizures mostly controlled. When I mentioned driving to my family doctor, he told me that people with controlled epilepsy are safer drivers than most.

13.

It's a wonder that I got in and attended university. University was on the other side of the city, and taking the bus took an hour and a half each way. I would sometimes have seizures on the bus and pass the university then I'd have to wait for the bus to come back so I could get off at the university; it would have been much better for me to live on campus.

Nonetheless I was going to university and working part-time at the Chrysler mini-van plant on the trim line. I was also taking fourteen pills per day.

Doctors were trying different medicine to see if they could control my seizures. How I managed going to university and passing – and working – on that much medication, is something only my higher power knows. It was a wonder that I could even attend.

While I was in university my uncle Don was seeing a girlfriend who was a nurse in Detroit, Michigan, and he told her about my case. She advised my uncle to send a letter about my case to Washington, DC to see if they could help. There was no internet or email in those days so I had to be patient waiting for the letter to reach Washington and then wait for a response. Roughly one month later I received a response notifying me of two Canadian doctors, one in Winnipeg, where I would have had no coverage and the other in London, Ontario where I had coverage.

My neurologist suggested that I finish university, set up an appointment at the hospital, and wait for a call (which could take years). At the time, my sister still lived in London, so I shared an apartment with her. Sharing an apartment with my sister was hard as we were opposites, she was experimenting with her sexuality and drugs with friends and I wasn't interested in that.

After five and a half months we got into a verbal fight and she said she was leaving and going to live elsewhere unless I moved out. Well, I found another place to live and was just about to move in when the hospital called with an opening. I ended up staying in the hospital for a few months for intensive evaluation of my problem.

I didn't know that this surgery was new, but it had just began the year before I had it done, so I was like a guinea pig, but it was my only hope to control the epilepsy.

During my stay at the hospital I had many EEGs (a test with flashing lights to read electrical activity in the brain) and an MRI (a test to detect structural abnormalities). This was a new test at that time, so I had to go to a different hospital in the city that had an MRI scanner. Doctors looked at the EEG results searching the wavy lines for spikes to see when they would occur. They wanted to figure out what triggered the spikes.

Once, the doctors tried to induce me into a seizure to see the spikes on the chart. I wasn't having a convulsion, so the doctors sent my mother home because they thought that her being with me was keeping me calm and preventing me from convulsing. She left, and the doctors thought it was my dad's turn to come to the hospital with me.

My room had no windows or sound, and the doctors thought this may help me to have a seizure. I thought that if I called my dad and said something that he wouldn't like his response would make me have a seizure.

It worked! The only problem was the stainless steel bars on the sides of the bed. When I did have a seizure it didn't register on the monitor because the bars were in the way! After the seizure, although my mother was half way home, she turned around and came back to the hospital.

I had hoped I'd be a candidate without needing the subdural surgery before the main surgery, but the EEGs and the MRI weren't good enough for the doctors to determine the source of the seizures, so the subdural surgery was required to help in finding the source (Epi-center) of the seizures. I had needles two inches into my head for two weeks. It was horrible. I could barely move my head on the hospital bed and it hurt badly, but I felt no matter how much suffering I had to endure, I wasn't going to live like this anymore.

After two weeks with the needles in my head they were finally removed and I was told I was a candidate for surgery. I was so happy, it seemed like there was hope after all.

Now I had to decide whether I wanted to have the auras gone or the falling down finished, tough decision. I decided to have the auras removed because it was a horrible feeling. I hoped that both issues would be resolved. My mother was with me most of the time at the hospital pre-surgery. My stepfather said it was okay for her to quit her job and stay with me during this time. My mother lived in Oakville and drove back and forth to London to be with me. Pre-surgery, I was told that the procedure had a 60% success rate and that I might be blind, have more brain damage or even end up dead afterwards. I felt I had no choice if I wanted a better life.

14.

My mother and stepfather were highly supportive of my decision to have the brain surgery, but my father was less so. He didn't want me to have the surgery because, at the time, I think he was scared. However, post-surgery when my father saw that I turned out fine (not mentally challenged), he had an attitude change and seemed happy about my decision.

Before the surgery I was tested and told I had a genius IQ in numbers, and as I was ecstatic. I felt like somebody finally knew I was good at something. Not just a mentally challenged person, as my doctor wrote years before. I was also told I was lucky it happened when I was young so the other side of my brain took over the functions that were damaged from epilepsy. During my research I came across an article stating that people with right temporal lobe epilepsy are not good at reading or directions, and they find it hard to locate new places. Well I don't fit this bill, as I am excellent with directions (east, west...), it is one of my strong points. I always love telling people how to get from point A to point B without getting lost. I even give them landmarks so they don't lose their way.

The following month I was booked for brain surgery (the main, eight hour operation) and had it done. The main surgery was hard as I had to keep my head still for eight hours; I began crying after an hour and the doctors won-

Shelley Kobelsky

dered if I was okay, I said "I just want to move my head", so they allowed me to move it a bit and then continued surgery. During surgery they asked me a question to ensure they were removing the right part of the brain, as I was awake. Right after surgery I had many seizures, one after another and the bed was shaking. Even the nurse was scared and asked my mother to help, as she had never seen anything like this before.

Immediately after brain surgery it's very important to walk, so you don't get a blood clot. My mother and the male nurses were trying to get me to walk but I wouldn't because I was in so much pain. The staff didn't know what to do, so my stepfather, Andy, walked over and said to me, "You don't want to hurt your mother, she's crying and worried about you; I'll help you get up and walk."

I got up and walked with him, looked at my mother and saw a big smile on her face, and then I managed to crack a smile. This moment was horrible because no one knew how I'd react post-surgery.

15.

Having brain surgery was a turning point for me.

I finally had hope that something had been done to control, or maybe even alleviate epilepsy. So, after the surgery I returned to university and did a paper on epilepsy.

My head had been shaved for the surgery, and I had little hair stubs. I wanted to wear a wig so it wouldn't be obvious, but then I thought about what would happen in a few months when my hair grew back? So, I dared to go to classes with a shaved head. Many students said they learned a lot about epilepsy and one person shared that she had epilepsy and grew out of seizures by the time she was seven. At the end of the course, a lady told me my head was cute shaven and that I looked good. This made me feel better. I graduated from university and would say that surgery has improved my life immensely.

Life post-surgery is another story. It's still abnormal, but I can feel fairly normal; hardly any seizures – just three since the day after brain surgery (I say this because I had some grand mal seizures as stated earlier, right after surgery). Hopefully, my convulsions won't come back on a daily basis ever again, as I must be under severe stress to cause one.

Post-surgery I've had a few seizures under extreme conditions. Once was when I walked for the first time after breaking my femur, I had one grand mal and one petit mal seizure. The other time was in an airplane right after my stepfather passed away, as I was close to him.

I always said – and still say – "I'm a human being" when I feel I'm not being listened to (ignored), whether with family or a close friend, when I feel comfortable enough. I get the sense that others don't want to hear me, thinking what they are about to say is more important.

In group situations, I would usually sit at the back of the room so that most people wouldn't notice me, and to this day I am still quiet in crowds. I never got over that!

After university in Windsor I had six part-time jobs at once, as there was a full-blown recession. It was tough to find a good job and I did what I felt I could to survive. My part-time jobs included security at a home for troubled teenagers on the midnight shift in a bad part of town. It was somewhat scary, my grandparents and mother hated me working at this place. They wanted me to quit but my father thought I should be working so I kept trying to get other work.

I later got transferred to a Transit Windsor yard and did security there, counting money in the US Tunnel bus at the end of the night and telling truck drivers, who were picking up cars, what time they needed to get to the Ambassador Bridge in order to clear customs. I was in a little a square building with windows. Again, the graveyard shift was a bit scary, but not like working at the troubled home where I was at the mercy of anyone hiding outside in the dark eerie grounds.

Finally I had enough and decided to move near Toronto where good jobs were easier to find. My stepsister loved me and wanted me to have a chance at the good life, so I got a job at the trust company where she worked, at their head office in downtown Toronto; it was a start. The human resources department tested me, they said I was the fastest person to do their test with no errors. While working there I got my own apartment in Mississauga and met a co-worker who became my best friend. We shared an apartment and I worked there for three and half years. We got a dog, something I had always wanted, so for eight months I had time with our dog.

I left that job under duress, it was beneath my skill-set. Again, I did it for survival as in the past. This was the beginning of me having a social network, which grew. After that job I tried selling new cars, that lasted six months. I met a boyfriend at my workplace and we tried dating, he was normal and cute. However one night we went out in downtown Toronto at the lake and he told me he wanted seven children, so after that I broke up with him as I didn't want any children. From zero-to-seven is a lot! I felt bad as he was an awfully nice person. However, I had my beliefs and I didn't want to hurt him by letting him think we would have children.

Later that year I joined a new corporation, helped get it going and developed it into a medium-sized company. So the following year my best friend and I purchased a townhouse in Mississauga which was close to my family and shared it for four and a half years. We decided to sell it as there was a high maintenance fee and a lot of structural work that needed to be done. My mother and stepfather had bought a new house in Cambridge, so I decided to buy from the same builder. I bought a new townhouse on the same street in Cambridge and moved in with my dog. Everybody on this street was from the Greater Toronto Area. I lasted three years and sold my townhouse. I then moved back to Mississauga since I was putting too many kilometres on my car and the winter could be brutal. I felt like a misfit in a regular neighbourhood with little kids; I didn't have any children or want to have any.

I was still trying to live a normal, happy life.

16.

The company I helped blossom and grow is still open today. When I started there I said it was my mission to take this company global with a family culture. We opened a Caribbean location, one in Alberta and another in British Columbia. The company later expanded to Montreal, Halifax and Newfoundland. I worked there for almost fourteen years.

The first few years of working at this company I felt was the new beginning of my life. I was the architect of my life for the first time and it was a great feeling. I could make my own choices, I had friends and close family I could share my life with. However, while working there, there were times I would experience dizziness, step down for a few minutes and continue working with a headache. I would do anything to keep the company growing.

I won an Achievement Award for being dedicated and motivated after ten years of service and I felt proud and happy.

A month later I broke my leg on the ice, so once again I lost control of my life. My life and work were never the same. I ran the company, had trust, and I was nicknamed the Warden. I felt like I had loyalty and respect. I carried many families' livelihoods, getting and keeping this going. The owners were immigrants and I felt like I was making many dreams come true. Even my family nickname is "Queen", I was like the Queen to them. Actually my uncle used to call me "Queen of the hyper" when I was three years old. He changed the lyrics of the song *Sweet Hitch-hiker* to *Queen of the Hyper*. Later, when I wasn't so hyper anymore I was called "Queen," which is still my family nickname today.

I was like "Donald Trump" in my family. I helped my family and had it all for about ten years. My work brought me joy. I got to use my organizational, creative and people skills. I loved making others feel comfortable and happy. I enjoy numbers and people, a great business person. Finally I decided to complete my rite of passage (confirmation) and it was right after a meeting in January in the parking lot I fell on the ice and broke my femur. I felt the devil stepped in, broke my femur, and this was the beginning of the end for me. I lost control of the company, and just like having epilepsy, I had to stay in hospital for a few weeks.

During my recovery, away from work, I was motivated to get my life back, I had to walk so the staff put me in the fast-track program. I ended in the hospital for about 20 days; pretty short for a broken femur bone. I then had physiotherapy for three months before I was deemed "back to normal".

Upon returning to work there was a new receptionist hired to help out and later other accounting people were hired and nothing felt right anymore. After working at this company for 13 and a half years, one day I walked into one of the owners' offices, fell over on a chair and was dizzy for a while. I was saying prayers in my head for strength to get me home. Well my prayers worked and I made it home safely.

I had done just about everything at this company except fixing and repairing the equipment that we began selling about three years after opening. I later stuck to accounting, keeping the numbers in order and enjoyed setting up our monthly open houses. I did many fun things during my time there but later I had a bad feeling in my stomach and I felt it was best to move on before I got really sick.

Epilepsy was no longer my greatest enemy. This time when I quit it was my choice, it wasn't epilepsy. However, I still end up with a personality of *having to overcome things* as a result of my epilepsy. I am presently a bookkeeper, and since I'm really good with numbers, employees from other locations will contact me if they need help with their reports and numbers.

17.

To this day, I am not good at interviews. Potential employers think I'm slow because of my delayed speech. Actually I'm the opposite of what I seem, as I am really quick and a genius in the numbers area. I love investigating numbers and license plate numbers. I am detail-oriented and analytical. I remember our phone numbers from the many places we grew up and I remember license plates, which comes in handy in some cases. I have been told a good career path for me would be politician, accountant, investigator or business owner. I've done all except a politician and I believe I would be an excellent forensic accountant, researching and investigating – my best skills.

The best advice I could offer anyone is to just do what you love – and remember: No matter how much you accomplish, when one huge strike happens – your Achilles heel – you can go down and out for the count. My life changed forever from falling on the ice and breaking my leg.

I never believed in a "career," I believe you just do a job. Do what you love and make a difference at it, whatever path you choose.

I've done so many types of jobs in my life and the only kind of job I have been told to avoid is anything with a lot of flashing lights or linear drawings – which I wouldn't be interested in doing anyway!

Almost a year into my new job I was let go. Once again I was called a misfit. I feel I have to keep going and that the dream job and life will come. I probably suffer from some sort of mental illness from all the suffering and name-calling I have endured. Even my genius IQ in numbers hasn't helped my potential, all because of my epilepsy.

Even Vincent Van Gogh, considered a genius as an impressionist painter, committed suicide from the depression that often comes with the harsh reality of living with epilepsy. I still question why I'm still alive. What's my purpose? I know I've taught many things and I accept people on their terms. This acceptance I believe comes from my experiences and what I've gone through. My mother has told me that I'm an inspiration to many, treading through rough waters and actually achieving some goals, persevering. No doubt many would have given up and not pursued the lifestyle they wanted. However, no matter what I accomplish I always feel I am not the woman I could have been – and I'm never quite sure of myself. This is the reality which isn't pretty; perhaps I could have been an Olympic swimmer had I not had the curse of epilepsy?

I have always believed that I could do and achieve many things, and with my Higher Power, I believe I have!

"Believe and receive. Doubt and do without!" That is one of my slogans! Another is: "If you're going to dream, dream big." No point in settling for peanuts. If you settle for peanuts you get monkeys. "Never fear, walk through it, you can do it."

18.

I finally met the man of my dreams, three years ago at a friend's barbeque. He is a "Road Scholar," one who has knowledge on various subjects through experience rather than via the educational system. He's greatly supportive and loving; just what the doctor ordered. Now we have lived together for about three years and are planning on getting married – absolutely exciting! As I mentioned, I don't want to have children and pass epilepsy on to the next generation, so I made sure that my partner didn't want children as well. I waited a long time and now I finally have a relationship in which each of us understands where the other is coming from. He still has daily challenges as well, so we help each other out to make life much better.

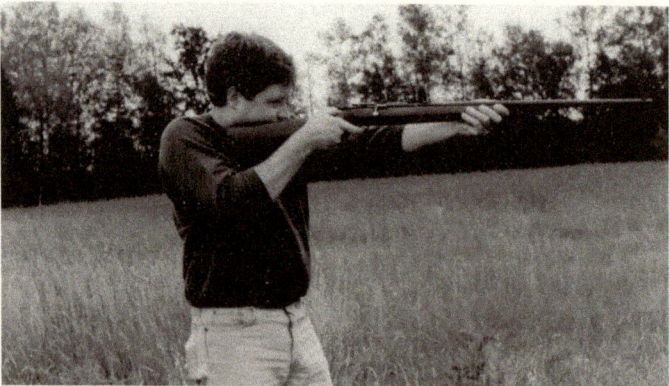

My fiancé Ken – a "Road Scholar."

Shelley Kobelsky

Life has its ups and downs, but now I have a partner to share my hopes and fears with.

My sister, Sherry, has become a poster person for the Canadian Mental Health Association and was featured in the *Windsor Star* to show how the mental health system today is still scattered and needs a lot of work. She currently volunteers at the Canadian Mental Health Association working at a diner. She has never been so happy. Her two boys are doing really well and things have finally come together with her new husband who has helped her so much. Sherry is also writing her story.

19.

I hope and dream that others will be touched by this story and that it will help people affected by epilepsy. I hope I have had an impact on the medical side as well, attempting to live first on all the medication, and then by having surgery.

Hopefully this will assist in seeking new treatments and cures for epilepsy. The secret is: "Don't give up! Persevere!" Have hope and keep plugging away as normally as possible. I always tried to beat it, moving on and finally we found an answer that solved 99.5% of the problem! I still take a minimal amount of medicine for epilepsy.

I just went to Buskerfest 2015, "Where fearless meets funny," in downtown Toronto. It's a fun few days in support of Epilepsy Toronto and the largest epilepsy event in the world, with street performers, acrobats and clowns from everywhere.

The final day features the *Purple Walk* for people with epilepsy. We donated money to assist Epilepsy Toronto and had many laughs there. While I was there I tried winning a prize, like I had years before. I hit the bullseye again (something I didn't see anyone else do while I was there!) but this time I didn't fall over afterwards. What a great feeling!

Hopefully research will continue and assist more

people, even transform the lives of patients. I believe sharing and being open with my story may help give others hope, knowing they can make it through even the most severe cases of epilepsy and live relatively normal lives.

I always felt guilty for not being able to participate in all the events, but in spite of my disorder I got to do most things. I believe we must be brave and persevere at all costs to make a difference and change the world for the better.

We are all going to die eventually, so we might as well try to live the best life possible!

If you see someone having a **seizure**, get an **adult** or call **emergency services** for help. If no adult is available, take the following steps:

- Remain **calm**

- Place the person on the **softest surface around** – a rug or sofa if you are inside, or the grass if you are outside

- Remove the person's glasses (if they are wearing any) and loosen any tight clothing

- Put something soft under the person's head, like a **pillow** or a **jacket**, and **lay the person on his or her side**. That way, if the person throws up, he or she won't choke on the vomit

- Do **NOT** try to restrain the person

- **Stay with the person** until he or she wakes up

www.ingramcontent.com/pod-product-compliance
Lightning Source LLC
Chambersburg PA
CBHW031134020426
42333CB00012B/375